Think W

– heralded by h
as a new cond
manage

"*This book is an absolute delight to read! It is written in a simple lucid manner, yet is packed with useful information, which will be particularly helpful to newly diagnosed diabetics and their families. Even those who have had diabetes for years will find this Pocket Guide invaluable in the management of their diabetes and their lifestyle - maybe it should have been called 'The Diabetic's Bible'.*"

Dr Chris Steele MB, ChB
GP and resident doctor on
ITV's 'This Morning' programme

"*The authors are very experienced in their fields. I have personally worked with Azmina, and an upbeat, practical attitude is very much her style. Complementing her skills with the inspiring thinking of a life coach like Nina, makes for a hearty cocktail of fun and knowledge.*"

Dr Hilary Jones MBBS
GP and resident doctor on GMTV

AN INSPIRATIONAL GUIDE
FOR PEOPLE WITH DIABETES

Think Well
To Be Well

by
Azmina Govindji
& Nina Puddefoot

with foreword by Dr Hilary Jones

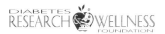

Staying well until a cure is found

Registered Charity No: 1070607
tel: 023 9263 7808   fax: 023 9263 6137
e-mail: drwf@diabeteswellnessnet.org.uk
website: www.diabeteswellnessnet.org.uk

Image on page 29: printed with kind permission of The British Meat Nutrition Education Service.

Published 2002 in the United Kingdom by:
Diabetes Research & Wellness Foundation™
Northney Marina, Hayling Island, Hampshire PO11 0NH
tel: 023 9263 7808   fax: 023 9263 6137
e-mail: drwf@diabeteswellnessnet.org.uk

Registered Charity No: 1070607

Printed by: Holbrooks Printers Ltd., Norway Road, Portsmouth, Hampshire, PO3 5HX

Price: £5.50 (UK)

ISBN 0-9537873-1-1

Diabetes Research & Wellness Foundation™…

…is an organisation dedicated to people with diabetes, their families, caregivers and healthcare professionals.

…has a mission to help find a cure for diabetes and to provide the support needed to combat the sometimes life-threatening complications of this debilitating condition.

…aims to keep people with diabetes *"Staying well until a cure is found"*.

To accomplish its mission…

DRWF provides funding for research into the causes, cures or alleviation of the complications of diabetes.

DRWF provides products to people with diabetes that enhance their knowledge and self-management skills.

DRWF promotes public education about the causes of diabetes, its prevention and treatment.

DRWF provides forums in the form of 'wellness' retreats, to establish confident self-management skills.

DRWF arranges exhibitions of diabetes products and services, for the benefit of those who live with diabetes.

Foreword

Whether you are newly diagnosed or have had diabetes for some time, knowing what to eat and being confident about your choices tends to be a struggle. With this book, these choices are made clear and simple. The facts about food are explained, such as how different foods affect blood glucose, how sugar acts in the body and why the fat story is significant in diabetes. Information is given in bite-sized pieces, which is far easier to digest, and this little guide gives you the basics, keeping the latest research and ideas very much in mind.

But the book goes further than this. Knowing what you should eat and then making those changes are two very different things. Most people know that smoking is bad for you, yet stopping smoking is a different matter. Most know that eating too many fatty foods makes you more prone to heart problems, but making the changes consistently isn't so easy. Flicking through these pages and catching the inspirational quotes and thought-provokers which touch at a deeper level, makes you think more closely about the choices you have in life and what's really important to you. The positive messages to eat wisely because you want to, not because you're being told to, are very empowering. And the facts are so cleverly summarised in the form of "Go Fishing" flow charts, that you can see at a glance how food and life choices can affect you and your health.

Reading this book reminds me of Aesop's fable of the competition between the wind and the sun to see which one could get a man to take off his coat. This book adopts the tone of the sun, that won the competition with warm and gentle persuasion. I wish this book had been available when my own son was diagnosed with diabetes at the tender age of seven.

The authors are very experienced in their fields. I have personally worked with Azmina some years previously on educational videos for diabetes, and an upbeat, practical attitude is very much her style. Complementing her skills with the inspiring thinking of a life coach like Nina, makes for a hearty cocktail of fun and knowledge.

Dr Hilary Jones MBBS

(Dr Hilary Jones joined the breakfast TV station, GMTV, where his sympathetic and laid-back style has made him a popular and respected medical opinion nationwide.)

Acknowledgments

The authors are indebted to DRWF for giving them the opportunity to unite their unique skills that began within regular newsletters and have culminated in the production of this inspirational book.

Both Azmina and Nina have aspired to sharing with the public their combined experiences and innermost thoughts on wellness, and this book represents the first of a series of publications from them. The authors therefore wish to express their eternal gratitude to the staff of DRWF, particularly Roslyn Elson, for putting faith and trust in them.

Special mention should also be made of those dear to the authors who have facilitated all the hours that went into the manuscript – Shamil, Bizhan, Shazia, Richard, and Nina's mum, Joan, who has first-hand personal experience of diabetes.

Contents

Contents (continued)

Contents (continued)

Contents (continued)

Preface

Readers of this book will notice an emphasis on foods and weight loss, interspersed with life guidance notes. This double-edged approach has a purpose – to stimulate an interest in changing to a healthier lifestyle, and to show how it can be done by altering how you think. And behind all of this is professional advice on the foods that can be eaten by people who have diabetes, and the dietary reasons that back up the advice.

The Diabetes Research & Wellness Foundation makes no apology for this approach, since the two questions asked over and again by so many people are – "How can I lose weight?" and (usually soon after diagnosis) "What can I eat?"

Type 2 diabetes (formerly called non-insulin-dependent diabetes and often referred to as late-onset or middle-age diabetes) comprises around 85-90 per cent of all the diabetes in the UK and throughout the world. This type of diabetes can begin by being overweight/obese and living a sedentary lifestyle, on top of having a genetic propensity for developing the condition. The charity recognises that people with type 2 diabetes will benefit most from this book.

The other form of diabetes – type 1 – was previously called insulin-dependent diabetes and is often referred to as childhood diabetes. This book is also relevant for people with type 1 diabetes, as the basic dietary and lifestyle messages are the same.

Other family members, carers, and – dare we suggest – even people without diabetes who simply wish to adopt a healthier lifestyle, will also find inspiration within the pages of this book.

Good health, fitness, and confidence in having personal control of your condition is essential to everyone with diabetes, no matter which type you have, so as to secure your health in the future.

Introduction

Making friends with your diabetes

This book is about a way of living life. It will inspire and empower you through helping you make good choices about your health. It will show you how your thinking and how adopting a positive mental attitude will irrefutably influence your overall sense of well-being, as well as add richly to other aspects of your life.

You will enjoy the 'thought provokers', and the up-to-date advice on food with the latest thinking on the diets for diabetes. Also, you will find health tips created with these dietary recommendations in mind – and recipes, all with a difference.

We believe that you'll find this little book is unique in its offerings.

Why me?

And so, you've just been diagnosed as having diabetes…

Whatever your situation, know that the way you eventually view your diabetes, the way you feel about the condition of diabetes (including the 'why me?'), will influence how you deal with your situation. By taking some simple steps to eat healthily and to monitor your diabetes regularly, you can live a full and active life.

We will invite you to check and challenge your thinking, approach and attitudes in relation to food choices and many other aspects of life, and show you that what you dwell on, you bring into existence. Your mental attitude is *your* responsibility. We will offer you ways in which you may choose to make changes.

Travel with us on a journey of discovery through these pages.

Chapter 1

*The most important product
of your life is you.*

Briefly, what is diabetes?

Diabetes occurs when the amount of glucose in your blood remains too high for too long because of irregularities or defects in your body's metabolic system. This damages the body's organs and tissues after a time.

To metabolise the foods we eat, our digestive system has to break down foods into their smallest constituents, such as sugars. Glucose is the simplest of all the sugars, made by the digestion of carbohydrate foods; other sugars are, for example, lactose (from milk products) and fructose (from fruits), but they all end up as sugar in our bloodstream.

We all need sugar for energy, and get most of it from starchy carbohydrate foods such as rice, bread, pasta, potatoes, and some from foods like sweets and chocolates (refined sugar).

A hormone from the pancreas, insulin, helps the glucose enter the cells of our bodies, where it is used as fuel. If you do not have enough insulin, or if your body resists the insulin you have (being overweight makes you more prone to this), then glucose can build up in your blood – with often unwelcome results.

The normal human body works on blood glucose levels of between 4 and 8 milli-moles of glucose per litre of blood (that means a normal blood glucose is 4-8 mmol/l).

In order to stay healthy for life, it is recommended that people with diabetes keep as close to this range as possible, and, in any case, try not to let their blood glucose exceed 10 mmol/l*.

* Diabetes Research & Wellness Foundation endorses these figures

If you have just been diagnosed with diabetes, make sure you get...

- A full medical examination.

- A consultation with a State Registered Dietitian to advise you on the right mix of foods for your diabetes.

- A consultation with a Registered Nurse or Diabetes Specialist Nurse to explain your individual treatment.

- Advice on driving, insurance, prescription charges and other general implications of diabetes.

- On-going education and assessment.

Chapter 2

*Good health, a sense of well-being
and a purpose for living
make any day beautiful.*

Acting like a lemon!

Here is something for you to try. Think of a lemon. See it in front of you and make the image as real and bright as you can. See it's colour clearly, and the small uneven grooves in the skin covering.

Now, in your mind's eye, run your finger along it, feeling the texture of its skin. With a knife, cut it in half. See the two halves side by side, and run your finger along one of the halves, feeling its moisture.

Lick your finger. Now pick up one of the halves and bite or suck it. Can you feel its acidic juices on your tongue?

Is there anyone who is not salivating yet?

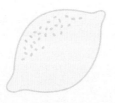

How did you do that?

You did it simply through your thoughts, which control the state of your mind, that in turn affects your body's response. In this case, it made your body's natural pharmacy kick in, providing the saliva that would be required in your mouth to eat a lemon. And it was done through your thoughts alone!

Imagine how this powerful and natural thinking can be used to influence your overall health and physical well-being. The mind is a phenomenal tool!

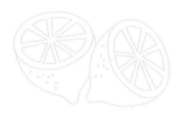

The mind-body link –
You are what you think

As you think it, so you become it!

And so you are constantly becoming your thoughts.

Changing your thoughts to experience a new positive mental attitude – for example, joy, happiness or peace – will allow the body to respond in a very different way, with a very different set of results.

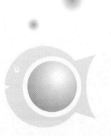

Act as if...

Here is an invitation.

Play with the belief that **every adversity has the seeds of at least equal benefit to you,** and that you can change the way you respond to anything in your life. Perhaps it is nature's way of teaching you things that you would not learn in any other way?

Your body receives its messages through your thinking and thence through the chemicals that your brain produces. Choosing a positive, resourceful state of mind is therefore essential to your overall state of well-being.

Laughing, loving, playing, choosing peace over conflict, acting out of gratitude and abundance, generally doing the things that you enjoy and spending time with the people you most value, are all ways of honouring yourself.

Thought provoker

Acting out of
well informed
choices today
will shape
your life
tomorrow.

Chapter 3

Make room for yourself in your life
by keeping it simple.

Healthy eating is
all about balance

There are lots of healthy eating tips in this book. It's a good idea to pick out the changes that you feel will fit easily into your lifestyle, choosing foods you enjoy.

Healthy eating is all about getting a balance – choosing a variety of healthy foods you enjoy and not forcing yourself to eat foods you dislike; balancing the protein foods and fat foods with the carbohydrates (starchy foods), vegetables and fruit in your meals in the correct proportions.

Use the information on the next pages to learn how.

The balance of good health

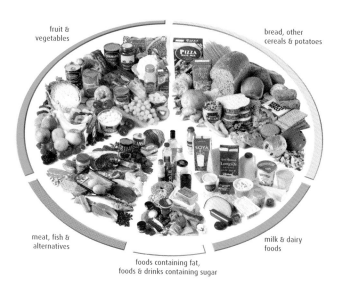

fruit & vegetables

bread, other cereals & potatoes

meat, fish & alternatives

foods containing fat, foods & drinks containing sugar

milk & dairy foods

A balanced diet uses something from each food group, in the proportions shown.

Good eating habits

- Eat regular meals.

- Gradually get to a healthy weight for you – and stay there (pages 78, 79 & 83).

- Choose foods with a low glycaemic index more frequently (page 104).

- Include fibre-rich foods.

- Include complex carbohydrate foods like pasta and wholegrains (page 32).

- Watch your intake of fried and fatty foods (pages 33 & 56).

- Eat five portions of fruit and vegetables a day (pages 34 & 35).

Swap high-sugar foods for low-sugar foods (page 43).

Eat more fish, and choose oily fish once a week (page 36).

Watch how much salt you use. Too much salt may be linked with high blood pressure.

Limit the amount of alcohol you drink (pages 96 & 97).

Avoid foods labelled 'diabetic'. They have no special benefit for people with diabetes and are generally no lower in calories and fat than comparable foods.

Starchy foods

Make starchy, carbohydrate foods (such as wholegrain breads and cereals or pasta) the main part of your meal.

Oat-based cereals like porridge and muesli are high in a particular type of fibre called soluble fibre, which makes them even more slowly absorbed than other starchy foods in general. They can play a significant part in keeping your blood glucose within a healthy range.

It is important to spread your intake of starchy foods evenly throughout the day, and to eat regular meals and snacks. This helps to reduce highs and lows in your blood glucose levels.

Fats and dairy foods

Since people with diabetes are at an increased risk of getting heart disease, watching and reducing your fat intake is particularly important. Foods high in saturated fat include full fat milk and cheese, fatty meats, lard, dripping, sausages, pies and pastries.

A range of spreads based on specific plant substances (called sterols and stanols) claim to help prevent heart disease by reducing blood cholesterol levels. These spreads can be effective as part of a low-fat diet, but note that they are only recommended for people with a raised blood cholesterol and not as a weight-reducing tool or as a spread for the whole family.

Guidelines for fat intake for an average-sized man or woman

Intake	Men	Women
Energy	2500 Calories	2000 Calories
Total fat	95 grams	70 grams
Saturated fat	30 grams	20 grams

Fruit and vegetables

Fruit and vegetables contain important vitamins and minerals that are needed for health, whether you have diabetes or not.

If you eat lots of fruit and vegetables, you are likely to be eating a healthy diet that provides more fibre, more anti-oxidant vitamins and less fat.

It is recommended that you eat five portions of these foods per day.

The anti-oxidant vitamins, beta-carotene (which is converted to vitamin A in the body) and vitamins E and C, have been linked to reduced incidences of heart disease, some cancers and some gut problems.

What is a portion?

1 medium fruit, eg an apple

1 large slice of melon or pineapple

1 cupful of strawberries or grapes

$^1/_2$ -1 tablespoon of dried fruit

1 small glass of fresh fruit juice

2 tablespoons of cooked or canned vegetables

A serving of salad

Meat, fish, nuts, pulses, and eggs

These foods are rich in protein, and many are good sources of vitamins and minerals, such as iron and zinc.

- Select lean cuts of meat and trim off visible fat.

- Remove the skin from poultry.

- Grill meat products such as sausages and burgers, and allow the fat to drain off.

- Eat fish twice a week. Drained, canned tuna in brine has half the fat of tuna in oil!

- Nuts are an important source of protein if you are vegetarian, and small amounts can help reduce blood cholesterol as part of a healthy diet.

- Pulses such as beans, sweetcorn, peas and lentils are an excellent source of soluble fibre.

- Eggs can be poached, boiled or scrambled instead of fried.

How to become your own best friend!

Becoming your own best friend means liking yourself for who you are!

Sometimes, when you are not at ease with aspects of yourself or your life, it can cause inner conflict and stress. Stress is responsible in some way for a variety of illnesses, even diabetes. To be ill at ease with yourself can be considered to be "dis-eased", not at ease.

There are some questions on the next page which may help you to choose what changes to make to enrich the quality of the relationship that you have with yourself, with those around you, and consequently with your life in general.

Living your life to its full potential is to embrace and recognise its true value as a precious gift.

Ask yourself...

How well do I fit in with my environments,
such as home, work and car?
What changes would you choose to make?

How do I communicate?
Are you truly being who you are, in your actions
and in what you say?

How fully do I express myself?
Are you utilising your natural talents, qualities
and skills in the way that you would most wish?

What do I most believe in and value,
and how do I show it?
What are you passionate about?

What makes me uniquely the person that I am?
How do you most wish to be thought of?

What value do I contribute to others,
including my community?
Why would others want to be with you
and spend time with you?

Thought provoker

Change your thoughts and you change your world.

Chapter 4

*You create your life
with each choice you make.*

Choices, choices, choices...

Eating is one of life's pleasures.

Knowing what is important for you, yourself, when selecting foods for you and the other significant people in your life such as your partner, children and family, will support you in keeping you motivated and on track with what you choose to eat and can eat.

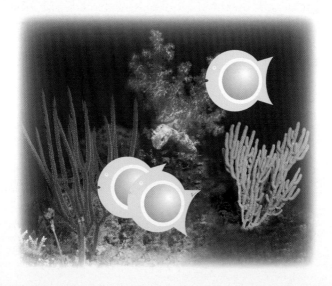

The truth about sugar

The effect a food has on blood sugar depends not only on how much sugar it contains, but also on a range of other factors like how the food is cooked, how mashed up it is, and what is eaten with it (see pages 104 & 105).

If you have a sugary drink on an empty stomach, your blood glucose will rise quickly. This is because the sugar in these drinks is absorbed into the bloodstream rapidly.

If a sugary drink is taken mixed with food, however, especially at the end of a high-fibre meal, the blood glucose rises more slowly because the sugar is digested along with the rest of the meal and not on its own.

Small amounts of sugar are fine for people with diabetes, but make sure you have it within an overall healthy eating plan and, ideally, at the end of a meal.

So, can you have your cake and eat it too?

To do both is your choice. But each choice you make will have its own set of results.

For example, choosing to have a bar of chocolate in-between meals will result in a rapid rise in your blood glucose. Choosing to have an apple instead will give you a different result – a slower rise in blood glucose – as well as vitamins and other nutritional benefits.

So, the choice you make about the chocolate will affect your blood glucose, which in turn will affect your diabetes, particularly if you make a habit of it!

Each choice will have a different consequence for you in terms of taste, calories and other things.

In the end – it's your choice, but you have to live with the consequences.

Waking up to conscious choices – a motivational tip

"When I become crystal clear about what is important to me about adopting and adapting to a healthy lifestyle, I increase my likelihood of succeeding."

You can support your thinking by finding a photograph of how you would like to look, one that expresses the 'new' you. By looking at it when you feel like straying, you will be reminded of what you can or want to achieve.

Consider making a list of all the benefits you will reap once you reach your goal, and keep the list near to hand.

Feedback – one of the currencies of life!

Your body is the ultimate feedback mechanism that you should listen to and pay attention to.

Here are a couple of examples –

If you have an episode of hypoglycaemia (a 'hypo' or low blood sugar) it can be embraced as a positive sign, as it will cause you to contemplate and change direction. So, for example, having a hypo at the same time each day or week gives you feedback that something (be it food, medication, stress, or exercise) needs to change. If listened to, it can nudge you in directions that will lead to improved care of your diabetes and greater happiness and health.

Or think maybe of a time when you indulged in perhaps one, two or three glasses too many – or in a spicy curry! How did you feel the next morning? Perhaps your head or stomach was feeding back to you in no uncertain terms that this was not very good for you!

When your mind or body is not at ease with something, you feel it through physical symptoms.

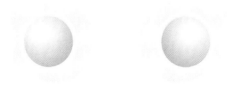

Today's choices become tomorrow's reality

Today's choices will make a difference to and contribute towards achieving what your life will be about tomorrow. What you choose today will shape your life tomorrow.

All aspects of your life, including your health, wealth, weight, self-image, home, work and relationships, are influenced by the decisions and choices that you are making now.

So, when you look at your physical body today, you'll know how your mind was thinking yesterday!

If you want to know how your body will look tomorrow, then examine your thoughts now!

Thought provoker

What's really important to you?

Is the choice that you are making right here and now taking you closer to achieving what's truly important to you? Whether it's the bar of chocolate or the apple, that extra glass of something or that éclair –

If you don't like what you've chosen, then choose again!

GO FISHING!

Do you have a sweet tooth?
If so, when are you likely to indulge?

Only with meals ～ This way the blood sugar levels are ～ more likely to be stable. Consequently you reduce the highs and lows in blood glucose, making your diabetes better controlled.

Between meals ～ This way, the blood sugar is more ～ likely to fluctuate from high to low. Consequently, you are more likely to have unstable blood glucose readings, which can increase your risks of getting complications.

When I'm feeling ～ Consequently, your meals and snacks ～ down in the dumps, may be less regular, leading you to or a tad under the perhaps making unhealthy food weather choices.

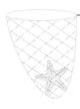

CATCH OF THE DAY!

~ You'll appreciate the high energy and an overall feel-good state, which also means the likelihood of a positive mental frame of mind!

~ Choose differently! Give yourself an extra boost of motivation. Think about the end goal – what it is that you really want – and direct your thoughts in that direction only!

~ Today's choices become tomorrow's future and that includes how you are choosing to feel. Think about supporting someone, in some small way. This way, you'll relieve yourself of the burden of self-obsession! By focusing on others, you'll feel uplifted and are therefore more likely to get back on track with your own goals.

Remember to throw back what you don't want and fish for what you do want!

Chapter 5

Fill your life with good company.

Happiness is within you

The most precious gift that you can give to another is to choose to be responsible for your own happiness and not put the burden of your needs at someone else's door.

Happiness is within YOU!

Through practice, you can learn to bring feelings of happiness into everything that you do, including your relationships. As you go through life happily achieving, wonderful experiences will follow.

Olive groves and orchards

The Mediterranean way of eating, with its abundance of olive oil, fish, nuts, fruit and vegetables, has been linked to a lower risk of conditions such as coronary heart disease and cancer.

The type of fat you eat has a significant effect on your health, and although the Mediterranean diet is relatively high in fat, the type of fat in it may be protective.

Most foods containing fat have a mixture of different types of fat, saturated through to mono-unsaturated, though one will generally predominate. Olive oil is classed as a source of mono-unsaturated fat.

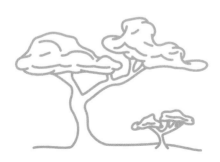

Getting your fats straight

- **Saturated fats** (found in butter, lard, processed foods, fatty meats, full-fat dairy products)

  These increase LDL (bad) cholesterol levels.

  Choose lean and lower-fat versions.

- **Mono-unsaturated fats** (found in olive oil, rapeseed oil, spreads made from these oils, nuts)

  These fats can help lower the bad LDL cholesterol levels and are thought not to affect HDL (good) cholesterol levels.

  Replace saturated fats with these wherever possible.

- **Omega-3 polyunsaturated fats** (found in oily fish like herrings, mackerel, pilchards, sardines and trout, and in linseeds and walnuts)

  These fats can help prevent blood clotting and help reduce another blood fat, tryglycerides.

  Eat more; aim for a serving of oily fish each week.

Omega-6 polyunsaturated fats (found in soya and sunflower spreads and oils, corn oil, grapeseed oil)

These fats can help lower the bad LDL cholesterol levels, but they are also thought to lower the good HDL ('protective') cholesterol.

Replace saturated fats with these, and eat in moderation.

Trans fats (found in hydrogenated spreads, processed foods such as biscuits, cakes, pastries)

Trans fats may raise the bad LDL in the same way as saturates, and are also thought to lower the good HDL. They may also lead to blood clotting.

Keep to a minimum.

Cholesterol (found in eggs, shellfish, liver, kidney)

Cholesterol in food has less influence over your blood cholesterol than saturated fats.

Eat in sensible amounts as part of an overall healthy diet.

The higher you can raise your HDL (protective) cholesterol, the lower your risk of heart disease becomes

Possibilities
and probabilities

There is enough evidence to suggest that, in life, if you think about possibilities you are very likely to turn them into probabilities. How you perceive the world and everything in it, will affect how your reality influences you.

A curious example is when someone believes he always catches three colds a year, and sure enough, that's exactly what happens – his name's on them! He is increasing the likelihood of turning this possibility into a probability just by believing in the probability; more so than another person who thinks "there are cold germs about" but does not entertain the possibility of getting infected.

Similarly, knowing that certain conditions exist which relate to the complications of diabetes, does not mean you have to help yourself to them!

Ignorance is (mental) poverty!

Enjoy making responsible choices and being accountable for your own life and its results. After all, you're driving your own bus!

True, it can feel quite scary being 'responsible', as then you can no longer lay the blame at someone else's doorstep or continue to find other reasons for why things haven't worked out for you.

To make responsible health choices for yourself you have to be informed. Grasping the concepts around diabetes may initially be difficult or seem impossible, and many people with diabetes leave it up to their healthcare professionals to guide them.

Perhaps taking responsibility for learning and understanding the facts that surround this condition, so that you can manage your own diabetes more effectively, would go a long way towards putting you back in the driving seat?

Hearty news

Your age, sex, genetic make-up and family history are outside your control. Once you accept this, then you can make excellent choices for keeping healthy and well, such as those offered here:

- Stop smoking.

- Aim to keep to a healthy weight.

- Replace saturated fats with unsaturated sources wherever possible.

- Eat five portions of fruit and vegetables every day.

- Replace salty processed foods with more unrefined foods.

- Eat oily fish once a week.

Make physical activity a regular part of your life or family life.

Incorporate some 'quiet time' into your daily routine.

Soluble fibre found in beans, lentils, peas, sweetcorn and oats can reduce blood cholesterol, so try to incorporate these foods regularly into your diet.

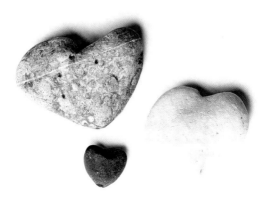

Circumstances don't make the man – they reveal him

You will already know that it is not always possible to have control over various areas of your life, including people and events, but remember – you always have control over how you interpret and respond to something in yourself.

Letting go of always having to be right, of anger, frustration, bitterness, resentment, jealously and all the other negative feelings that prevent you from continuing on the path of least resistance towards your goal, will make an instant difference to your state of inner peace.

Mental flexibility is the key here.

Make it a family affair

Going it alone is certainly possible, though you might like to involve the rest of the gang in your new lifestyle. Supporting each other has lasting benefits.

Even making meals doesn't have to mean cooking a different meal just for you. Get everyone involved in this healthier way of eating. Changing your cooking oil and adding some extra vegetables often goes unnoticed. Maybe the only thing that will get noticed is the delicious aroma of those Mediterranean garlic and herbs – and possibly requests for second helpings!

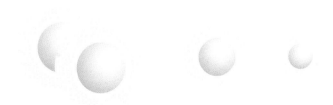

It's your life

Gaining the support and love of those closest to you has an incredible influence.

Choosing to spend time with those who nurture and nourish your values will help you to attain your goals. Mix with messy people and your life could become messy; mix with happy people and you'll learn about happiness.

Spend your time with people who enjoy looking after their health, and guess what happens?

Take advantage of joining groups of positive people coping with their diabetes.

How do you find yourself thinking about your diabetes?

To think " I am a diabetic", implies that you have allowed the condition to be a part of your identity, who you are, as opposed to what it really is – a medical condition. It controls you.

Thinking of it instead as a manageable condition, enables you to control it through self-empowering choices, with optimism and dignity.

GO FISHING!

 Are you conscious of the types of fat you eat?

I choose foods and cooking methods which are low in fat	As part of an overall healthy lifestyle, these foods help you keep in shape and help your diabetes and general health.
I eat oily fish once a week	The special omega-3 fats in oily fish have been shown to be protective against heart disease, a classic complication of diabetes. Consequently, choosing oily fish weekly simply reduces your risks!
I eat fatty meats and full fat dairy products because I can't resist them	It's fine to choose these foods; just watch how often. If you overdo such high animal fat foods, you are more likely to gain weight and are also more prone to raised blood cholesterol.

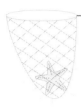

CATCH OF THE DAY!

~ Acting out of these well-informed choices today will shape your life tomorrow. Remember that life is like a building process – it has an accumulative effect.

~ Celebrate your choice here and keep reminding yourself of the rewards that this brings!

~ If your sense of health and wellness is not what you would wish it to be – then doing and eating as you've always done can only get you more of the same results. If you don't like what you're experiencing, change it, NOW!

Remember to throw back what you don't want and fish for what you do want!

Red lentil and carrot soup

Heat two teaspoons of vegetable oil and fry a chopped onion, 2 diced carrots and a bay leaf for a few minutes. Stir in 500ml of hot vegetable stock and 100g (3$^1/_2$ oz) dried red lentils. Return to the boil, cover and simmer for about 15 minutes until the lentils are cooked but not mushy.

Stir well, add more hot water if necessary, season and mix in 2 tablespoons of freshly chopped coriander leaves.

Pour into warmed bowls and serve with warm crusty bread.

[Serves four.]

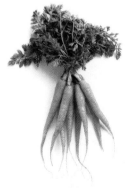

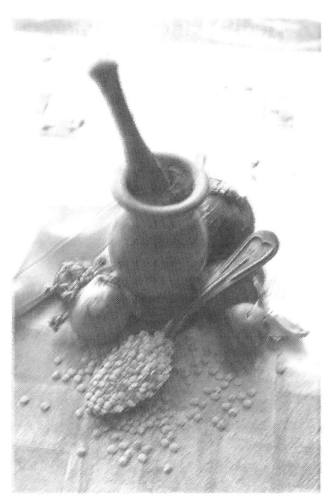

Raspberry and cream towers

For two towers you will need 6 small sheets of filo pastry, 125g (4½oz) each of half-fat crème fraiche and fresh raspberries, and 2 teaspoons of icing sugar. Preheat the oven to Gas 4/180°C/350°F. Cut 6 circles of filo pastry, each around 10cm (4 inches) in diameter. Line a baking tray with parchment paper and then place the circles on top. Dust them with icing sugar and bake for about 5 minutes.

Once cooked and cooled, lay one circle onto a dessert plate and top with a generous teaspoonful of half-fat crème fraiche and then a layer of sliced fresh raspberries. Place another filo circle on top and repeat the layers. Dust a final layer of pastry with icing sugar, and repeat for the second tower. Puree any remaining raspberries and drizzle this around the dessert.

Serve immediately.

[Serves two.]

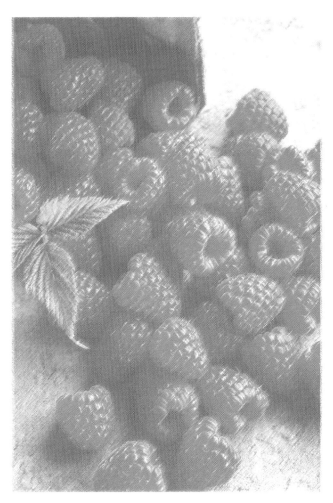

gettyimages/Joe Felzman

Chapter 6

> *Your beliefs are your reality.*
> *If you don't like the reality you see,*
> *change your beliefs!*

Weighty matters

Without the 'right' thinking, approach and attitude, the best slimming plans in the world are unlikely to work!

Why do most diets only last an hour and a half (just kidding, although in some cases this would be true!)? The answer is quite simply that your mind will always opt for the easiest route. Interpret something as being difficult or painful and your mind will wonder why on earth you would want this, and revert to what it interprets as being pleasurable – hmmm… another chocolate bun! – thus inadvertently sabotaging your goals in the process.

By changing your thinking to *interpret your goal as being fun and easy*, you are far more likely to achieve your goal.

How do you shape up?

If you are 'apple-shaped', you have greater health risks than if you are 'pear-shaped'. Check if you are carrying too much weight around your middle. Are you…

A man with a 37 inch or more waist?

A woman with a 32 inch or more waist?

Your Body Mass Index (BMI) tells you whether you are of a desirable weight for your height. To calculate your BMI, take your weight (in kilograms) and divide this by your height (in metres) squared.

$$\text{BMI} = \frac{\text{Weight}}{\text{Height}^2}$$

The most desirable range for all people is a BMI of between 20 and 24. If you need to lose weight, men can often do so on 1500-1700 Calories per day, and women on around 1200 Calories per day.

Energy flows where attention goes

"Don't think about kangaroos!"

At this moment, you will find you can't *not* think about kangaroos. The conscious mind finds it a stretch to hold a negative command, and so deletes it.

Or, tell a child… *"Don't spill your drink!"*

The chances are that that's exactly what will happen – the child will spill the drink. In addition to deleting the negative command, the mind also works on the last instruction received, which in this example is effectively a command to spill the drink.

This explains how it is that, if you tell yourself not to overeat, drink, smoke or worry, (to name but a few), the more you will do it! In the above example, a better result would be achieved by asking the child to *"Hold the cup tight!"* rather than telling him or her not to spill the drink.

If you keep thinking about what it is that you DO want (instead of what you don't want), then you are increasing your chances and the likelihood of achieving it.

With a little practice, you can begin to achieve the results that you really want, simply by being mindful of how you are thinking.

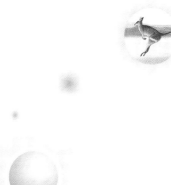

Pain versus pleasure

In the short-term many people opt for instant gratification, but this is sometimes at the risk of creating long-term pain for themselves.

Let's consider an example. Someone wishes to lose a few extra pounds. The long-term benefits are obvious to them – they would feel better about themselves, their clothes would fit better, their self-confidence would increase, and overall they would feel healthier and more energetic.

How interesting is it then that that same person will think up a multitude of reasons to put off even getting started!

Keep the irresistible, attractive image of the 'new you' uppermost in your thoughts, and remember the feel-good benefits of good health and the well-being that goes with it.

Successful slimming

A healthy way of eating, tailored to your needs, may not sound as attention-grabbing as quick-fix diets, but the evidence is that this is the best way of becoming slimmer sensibly and of keeping the weight off.

State Registered Dietitians can advise you on appropriate strategies to get to your target weight slowly but steadily.

Food tips for weight control

Have regular meals, preferably of a similar size each day. Don't miss meals.

Fruit and vegetables can help fill you up.

Bake, grill, roast without fat, microwave, steam, poach, char-grill, stir-fry and griddle instead of frying foods.

Have to hand some nibbles such as carrots, chopped fruit, sugar-free drinks or a mug of low-calorie soup.

No pain, no gain?

So what is the first step in making a change?

Start by choosing to overcome your problem – and mean it!

Think of the analogy of going to the gym. You wouldn't expect the perfect body after working out for just one session, would you? Similarly, you cannot train your mind in only one session of new thinking. You need to keep reinforcing it through repetition, just as you would your physical body in the gym if you wanted that new figure.

Willpower boosters

Put up a photograph of yourself before you gained weight. It will remind you of what you can achieve.

Weigh yourself only once a week.

Set realistic targets, such as a loss of 5-6 pounds in a month. Reward yourself with a trip to the theatre or a new book when you reach your target.

Make a list of all the benefits you will have once you reach your goal.

Eat on a smaller plate to make your meals look bigger.

Brush your teeth often to help you avoid those unnecessary extra mouthfuls between meals.

Eat at a table and be conscious of what you're eating.

Distract yourself when you feel like over-indulging.

Helpful questions
to ask yourself

What is truly important to me
about succeeding with this goal?

How will achieving this goal make me feel ?

How much more could I go on to accomplish
(in other areas of my life)?

How could others benefit if I make this change?

How much happier will I feel?

Understanding indulgences

There may be several reasons for an over-indulgence – comfort, security, boredom, habit, feeling 'down', hunger, social reasons, or to help you cope with stress or unpleasant feelings.

However, continuing to feed the habit will only reinforce the effect it's having. Looking for healthier ways to have this same need fulfilled will be of greater overall benefit.

What would have to happen for your need to be met in a healthy and functional way?

Your 'healthy and functional' response could be: taking up a hobby that would truly interest you; exercising; learning something new that would bring you great enjoyment; or developing (even more) fulfilling relationships.

Steps to success

When you are crystal clear about why you would like to have a healthier lifestyle, you will increase your chances of success through having a lasting motivation to succeed.

- What will having this new lifestyle do for you?

- How will having this new image affect your confidence, work performance, social life and belief in yourself?

- How will it affect the way you interact with others – family, friends and colleagues?

Once you know the impact and benefits the new lifestyle will give you, the energy with which you move towards your goal will be vastly multiplied. You can then take this learning to other goals you want to achieve…

Are you willing to begin the journey?

Let's get physical!

Physical activity helps your body to release endorphins – natural painkillers – which can in turn help you combat stress and feel energised.

Incorporate simple activities into your daily lifestyle and gradually work up to 30 minutes of activity five times a week.

Use the stairs instead of the lift; run up and down steps; walk at a pace that leaves you slightly breathless.

Take up a sport that you enjoy. Swimming with the kids or line-dancing classes with a friend can be a fun way of working out.

Remember that activity can be therapeutic, so tackling those garden weeds can have more benefits than you think.

Yoga has a strong relaxing and calming effect, besides being a safe and gentle way of exercising.

Uplifting your mood

Exercise is linked to brain function. The more regular exercise you do, the better your brain performs. Self-esteem increases, endorphins enhance your mood and promote that general 'feel-good' factor.

When you make a conscious effort and exercise, your tolerance to pain increases, as does your positive mood.

Muscle relaxation after exercise reduces tension levels and eases your nervous system, which helps get rid of pent-up energy and tension. This also promotes natural healing.

Interestingly, there is a strong link between exercise and mental health. People who take regular exercise are less likely to suffer from depression, and those suffering from depression can reduce their symptoms through exercise.

It's all win-win.

Thought provoker

Living up to your own true sense of identity is probably one of the most powerful forces to support you in making important changes.

Who you perceive yourself to be and what fits in with that perception will drive this.

You can't run away from yourself!

GO FISHING!

 When you're watching your weight, what do you do?

Mostly, I eat regularly and in small amounts and I aim for a slow steady weight loss. I really only eat when I'm hungry

~ A weight loss of 1-2lb per week is the best way to ensure that the weight stays off! Eating regular small meals is also good for your diabetes.

I'm currently making gradual changes to my lifestyle – foods and regular exercise

~ A tailored approach is great – the sure way to becoming slimmer is to choose a plan that fits in with your current lifestyle. Team this up with regular physical activity and you've got it made!

I often try crash diets and milk shake diets as they promise quick results!

~ There is no healthy way to lose weight fast. Such diets encourage a dieting mentality and yo-yo dieting is more harmful to your health than being slightly overweight.

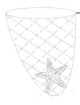

CATCH OF THE DAY!

~ You'll appreciate a state of consistent high energy and a sense of overall well-being which will help you to sustain a positive mental attitude. This is likely to support you in reaching and maintaining your ultimate weight.

~ You've done the trickiest part! You're making important changes, today. The choices that you make now will shape your life. In addition, perhaps you can find a new interest in some aspect of your life that will truly fulfill you.

~ Change your thinking to interpret your goal as becoming pleasurable and fun. Let it become an enticing way of enriching your life. This way, you're likely to succeed long-term, as opposed to the quick fix methods that don't necessarily last!

Remember to throw back what you don't want and fish for what you do want!

Chapter 7

Every time you let go of something limiting,
you create space for something better.

Alcohol

Alcohol is not out of bounds just because you have diabetes. The key is to drink sensibly and to balance it with food, and make the right choices – for you.

The life choices that you make in any precious moment in time become another brick in the building process of your life – your body, of course, acting as your mirror in what it reflects back. Should you indulge in those two or three glasses too many, you can usually count on your body letting you know – sometimes in no uncertain terms, through puffy eyes, a headache, or a fragile stomach the next morning!

So even if you have diabetes, there's no reason why you can't enjoy an occasional drink or even a small regular drink, unless of course you have been advised to avoid alcohol for another medical reason.

Safe drinking

The maximum recommended daily limit for men is 3-4 units per day and for women is 2-3 units per day. It is advised that people with diabetes keep well below these maximum limits.

Alcohol can cause hypoglycaemia. Drinks that are higher in alcohol content (such as spirits) are more likely to cause this. Therefore avoid drinking on an empty stomach and always have something to eat when drinking, also afterwards.

If you enjoy spirits, try to use the sugar-free/ slimline mixers.

One unit of alcohol is equal to:

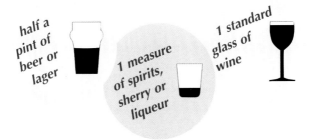

half a pint of beer or lager

1 measure of spirits, sherry or liqueur

1 standard glass of wine

What will having this drink do for me?

This is perhaps one of the key questions to ask yourself when you are tempted by alcoholic drinks, especially if you are about to reach for yet another one that is likely to take you beyond your limit.

Drinking is commonly associated with the need to feel more relaxed, especially in social circumstances, as it is with stress or comfort.

You may wish to explore what it is that you really get out of drinking. What need does it meet that is not being met in any other way?

Like any habit, a drinking pattern CAN be broken – by interrupting it.

So make a conscious effort to distract yourself by (for example) moving around. Any change in your physiology will have a considerable influence on your thinking. Consider going for a walk, taking a bath, doing some housework, cooking, reading or make a phone call.

You get the picture?

Drinking slowly is also a good tactic.

If you are in a pub, you could get up and go to the toilet, or go and speak to someone, or have a game of snooker or darts. Do anything that temporarily takes your mind off drinking. The chances are that, if or when the thought returns, it will have less temptation for you and you will be more likely to let it go.

Thought provoker

How are you directing your energy and thoughts when you think about alcohol?

How could you now direct your energy, knowing what you know?

For example, "I choose sound health".

Chapter 8

Your beliefs select the reality you see.

Trust the process

Choosing the path of wellness requires you to look for all the good things that already exist in your life, despite life's adversities.

One person may notice the glorious scenery visible out of the window, and another might choose to pay more attention to the dirty pane of glass.

You can choose to have preferences in your life and still be grateful for what shows up! Learn to trust what is happening in your life at any given moment, even if you don't yet know its purpose.

A story

A father and his son owned a farm. One day the only horse that they had ran away.

"What terrible, bad luck", the neighbours cried.

"Good luck, bad luck, who knows?" said the farmer.

Several weeks later the horse returned, bringing with him three wild mares.

"What excellent luck", said the neighbours.

"Good luck, bad luck, who knows?" replied the farmer.

The son began to ride the wild horses and one day he was thrown and broke his leg.

"What bad luck", said the neighbours.

"Good luck, bad luck, who knows?" replied the farmer in his enigmatic manner.

The following week the army came to the village to take all the young men to war. The farmer's son was still disabled with his injury and so was spared.

Good luck, bad luck, who knows?

The latest thinking

The latest recommendations on diabetes incorporate glycaemic index (or GI) as a logical approach to understanding and interpreting how different foods affect blood sugar.

GI is a ranking of foods by numerical value dependent on how rapidly the food reaches the blood as glucose. The faster a food is broken down during digestion, the quicker will be the rise in blood glucose, and the higher it will remain. Foods that cause rapid, high blood glucose levels are given appropriately high GI numbers (above 70).

'Whole' foods such as whole grains, and those high in 'soluble fibre' such as lentils, will take longer to be broken down by the body and will thus cause a slower rise in blood glucose and lower blood glucose levels. Foods like this are given low GI numbers (below 55). Foods with values between 55 and 70 are 'moderate GI' foods.

Just imagine how easy it is to digest hummus. Hummus is already in small particles, so the body doesn't need to mash it for too long before it is digested and ready to go into the bloodstream as glucose.

Now try to imagine digesting a casserole containing whole chick peas – how much longer that will take. Whole chick peas will slow down the rise in blood glucose much more than pureed hummus. This is the case with most whole foods – compare a whole lentil curry with pureed lentil soup, or a jacket potato with mashed potatoes, or granary bread with white bread.

Foods with a high GI, such as sugar-rich breakfast cereals, French-fries, full-fat dairy cheeses, are not "bad" foods. Keep an eye on how often you eat them and serve them with healthy accompaniments.

To use GI intelligently, choose to buy foods with a low GI regularly. Low GI foods in a meal will lower the impact of any high GI foods in the meal.*

The key to healthy eating is to get the right mix of foods.

* For more information on GI, see resources on page 127.

Remember to fly smart

Have you ever watched a moth that, time and time again, keeps banging against the windowpane or light bulb trying to get to the light? Unless it changes its approach, the results will remain the same!

How does this relate to making right choices?

By changing your approach and making a conscious decision to change (say) the foods you select and the meals you eat, or your 'couch potato' way of life, you will get what you set out to achieve, be it reaching and maintaining your optimum weight or having that feel-good factor of wellness.

Be a smart moth!

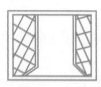

Food for thought

Decide what it is that you really choose.

Do something about it – take action!

Notice what's working and what's not, and use this as a feedback mechanism to yourself.

Keep changing your approach (don't be like the moth!) until you start to achieve.

Find ways of maintaining your healthier way of eating by reminding yourself of what you can achieve.

GO FISHING!

 How do you choose your foods?

I seek out and choose foods with low GI (see page 104) as often as I can

~ Consequently, you are making excellent choices for a steady blood glucose, one of the most important aims of treatment of diabetes. ~

I make food choices irrespective of the GI content

~ Consequently, you are being less aware of the effects different foods have on your diabetes and your blood glucose, making it more difficulty to keep in check. ~

I choose foods that are high in GI because I like them more

~ Consequently, your blood glucose levels are more likely to be unstable. ~

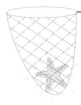

CATCH OF THE DAY!

~ Congratulations! Making these kinds of conscious choices will enrich your life through a sense of achievement, which in turn is likely to keep you motivated and up-beat in your mental approach and attitude.

~ Ignorance is mental poverty! This could have direct consequences related to your health. Enjoy finding out about the choices that exist and take responsibility for your life and its results. After all, you're in control!

~ You can start by choosing differently today and make your life richer by consciously choosing wellness. Short-term, many will opt for instant gratification, but this can be at the risk of creating long-term issues for themselves. Make up your mind to make the change here and now and then stick with it!

Remember to throw back what you don't want and fish for what you do want!

Thought provoker

Choice: If I continue to behave,
eat and think in ways that I've always
done, then I'll get what I've always got!

If you don't like what you've chosen,
then choose again!

Chapter 9

> *Every day, in every way, I am getting better.*

The balancing act

Life is all about balance. Acquiring balance in ALL aspects of your life is to live your life in a state of wellness.

Ill health comes from being out of kilter, but good health returns when you pay attention to your mental, physical and spiritual well-being.

Making meals

Making healthy meals is not a life sentence; it's a way of ensuring you make the right choices today that will shape a better future for you tomorrow.

But tomorrow seems so far away. Not so when you know that the accumulative effect of today's choices is tomorrow's results!

Having diabetes means that you *can* enjoy a variety of tasty foods based on your current condition and treatment.

Although what you eat is best tailored to your needs with the help of a specialist dietitian, the sample menu plan that follows will give you ideas on the types of foods for anyone wishing to keep to a healthy lifestyle, whether or not you have diabetes. The actual amounts have not been included as recommended amounts vary from person to person.

Sample Menu Plan

Breakfast

Small glass of unsweetened fruit juice, or fresh fruit;

Fibre-rich breakfast cereal, e.g. muesli, branflakes, wheat biscuits, porridge;

Semi-skimmed or skimmed milk;

Wholegrain, white or brown bread;

Unsaturated margarine or low-fat spread;

Reduced-sugar jam or pure fruit spread.

Mid-morning

Oat or wheat-based biscuits, preferably reduced-fat, or fresh fruit.

Lunch

Wholegrain bread, pasta, rice, potatoes (preferably whole and with the skin), pitta bread or chapatis;

Reduced-fat main meal, such as chicken or turkey, lean ham, drained tuna in brine, beans (e.g. baked beans, mixed bean salad), reduced fat cheese (e.g. half-fat cheddar, Brie, low-fat soft cheese) or a little full-fat cheddar cheese (grated goes further), boiled egg, etc.;

Mixed salad with fat-free dressing or reduced-calorie mayonnaise, or a large portion of vegetables;

Fresh or dried fruit.

Mid-afternoon

Plain biscuits, a few nuts and raisins, low-fat diet yoghurt, or fresh fruit.

Dinner

Rice, pasta, potatoes, etc as lunch;

Lean meat, fish, egg, cheese or pulse vegetables cooked in the minimum amount of fat;

Mixed salad or large portion of vegetables;

Fruit-based dessert, such as raspberry and cream towers (*see page 74*), or fresh fruit, low-fat diet yoghurts, a scoop of ice cream, or canned fruit in natural juice.

Eat well to be well

So, what are the chances of you truly enjoying your food, and experiencing the pleasures of every mouthful? Think about balance, and remember you always have a choice in the foods you eat.

Eating well will have positive effects for you, both mentally and physically.

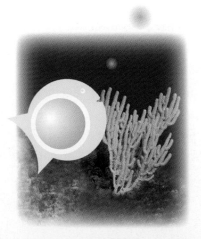

Old habits die hard

Old habits die hard, or so you may have heard.

Not so!

Change can happen in an instant if you are determined to make the change. It's deciding to make the change that can take longer. In other words, the more you use that same and familiar pathway, the more habitual your response becomes.

If you want to change something, then stop conditioning it! Lose it, don't use it! In this case, that's exactly what you want to do – lose those old habits!

Making it work for you

Knowing and choosing what you want to work for you, is making a true commitment towards achieving the result that you want.

Consider, even as you read this, what it is like to see yourself eating the healthiest foods, knowing the positive effects and influences that this is having on your body. Perhaps acting out of this picture encourages new and different actions, including whatever you choose to put into your picture!

As a direct result of following this outcome, see (just as an example) your glucose levels balancing perfectly. What feelings of well-being does that evoke in you?

Remember – think well to be well!

Your future in your hands

By choosing to adopt a healthy way of eating and living, getting the information and guidance you need and being responsible for your diabetes and your health, you will be able to achieve an improvement in your blood glucose levels, your overall health, your life, and thereby improve your risk of later complications.

Start from where you are today, here, now.

Yesterday and the past is the torn-up cheque – it's been and gone! Today gives you a fresh start, and the decisions and choices that you are making now will shape what you have tomorrow.

Wellness is not just about what you eat, it's also about what you do and how you think – and that means exercising, taking responsibility for your diabetes, and always being alert to your mental processes.

Starting today

You can start by focusing on what you can do TODAY to make your life richer, and of course this includes improving your health and well-being.

You can consciously choose wellness – today. As you think it, so you become it!

Whatever and whoever you have become, it is due to the cumulative thoughts that you have about yourself, about who you are. Your responses are a result of how you think of yourself, and your actions will be consistent with your thoughts around your identity.

In other words, your identity governs your actions.

Before you adopt a new way of eating or exercising, it is advisable that you speak to a dietitian or medical advisers.

If you have not yet seen a dietitian, you can ask your doctor to refer you to a State Registered Dietitian at the local hospital or community centre.

A number of leisure centres accept referrals onto exercise programmes from a doctor.

Thank you!

As you now come close to the end of this book, it only remains for us to thank you for sharing this inspirational and educational journey with us.

Knowing that you always have control over your thoughts, which govern your feelings and lead to your responses, you will know that despite life's little tests and challenges along the way, you are your own very special best friend.

As with any precious friendship, we hope that you will choose to nourish and nurture it and place it in your best light. You owe it to yourself.

Feed a man a fish and he eats for a day.
Teach a man how to fish and he eats for life.

My Achievements

*Jot down your successes here, and refer to
this list whenever you need a boost.*

Resources/Information/Advice/Support

BOOKS

Great Healthy Food – Diabetes, by Azmina Govindji. Published by Carroll and Brown, 2001.

The Glucose Revolution (formerly The GI Factor), by Dr Anthony Leeds, Professor Jennie Brand Miller, Kaye Foster-Powell and Dr Stephen Colagiuri. Published by Hodder and Stoughton, 1996.

Quick and Easy Cooking for Diabetes, by Azmina Govindji, Published by Harper Collins,1997

Diabetes Weight Loss System, by Professor Walter Bortz, Sharon Bortz and Patricia Mathis. Published by DRWF, 2000.

INFORMATION LEAFLETS – free from DRWF

- Facts about diabetes
- Looking after your eyes
- Looking after your feet
- When you are ill
- Injection insulin – sites and swellings
- Impotence – what you should know

The Diabetes Wellness Network™ – a supportive network set up by the DRWF. Members receive free a monthly newsletter and pocket diary.

Diabetes Wellness Retreats – residential events organised by the DRWF, where people with diabetes listen and talk to the professionals, as well as meet other people with similar diabetes conditions to themselves.

'Active With Diabetes' holidays – DRWF arranges safe, gentle, short walking holidays in collaboration with Ramblers Holidays Ltd. Each holiday has one or more diabetes professionals in attendance at all times. An excellent way of experiencing how to remain active.

Information on all DRWF leaflets, publications and events can be obtained from the charity direct. Ask for a free diabetes alert necklace.

If you have enjoyed reading this book
and would like to find out more
about Az & Nina's other publications
or courses, they can be contacted at:

Steps 4 Life
tel: 01273 305 733
fax: 01273 305 933
e-mail: nina.puddefoot@btinternet.co.uk